Honoring My Temple

Daily Devotionals for Changing Your Eating Habits with God at the Center

Honoring My Temple
Written by Kelly Wenner

For permission requests, contact:
SoulStrength Fit
www.soulstrengthfit.com

ISBN: 979-8-9929143-3-7

Table of Contents

Welcome to Honoring My Temple

Daily Devotionals for Aligning Your Health and Nutrition with God's Purpose

God has given you an incredible gift—your body. It's not a temporary or unimportant part of who you are, even though it's often treated that way. Some Christians view the body as separate from their spiritual lives, as if it doesn't matter in their relationship with God. Meanwhile, the culture around us often sends the opposite message—treating the body as if it's the most important thing about us. But neither extreme reflects the truth.

As followers of Christ, we are called to be His ambassadors here on earth—and our bodies are the vessels through which we live out that calling. God gave us our bodies for a reason. He has a plan for how we care for them, and a design for our health that reflects His wisdom and love.

In a world that constantly pulls us in opposite directions, it's easy to lose sight of what's true. But your worth is not defined by how you look or by the world's standards of beauty. Your body is a tool to live out God's calling with strength, joy, and endurance.

Honoring My Temple is more than a devotional about physical health; it's an invitation to align every part of your life—including your nutrition, fitness, and self-discipline—with God's design. Throughout these devotionals, you'll explore how properly caring for your body is an act of worship, how self-discipline is a fruit of the Spirit, and how small, intentional choices can lead to lasting changes.

This journey is not about striving for perfection—it's about surrender. It's about learning to steward your body well, not through rigid rules but through wisdom, gratitude, and reliance on God's strength. My prayer is that this devotional will encourage you, challenge you, and inspire you to care for your body in a way that honors the One who created it.

For a deeper experience that strengthens both body and spirit, consider pairing these devotionals with the *Honoring My Temple* faith-based fitness workout program from SoulStrength Fit. This program includes faith-centered workouts that correspond with the devotionals, encouraging growth in both physical health and spiritual focus. Visit www.soulstrengthfit.com to learn more.

Let's begin this journey together— pursuing health, strength, and a deeper connection with God as we honor our temples for His glory.

Introduction: Learning to Eat Mindfully

Introduction Learning to Eat Mindfully

"May my meditation be pleasing to him, as I rejoice in the LORD."
— Psalm 104:34 (NIV)

Mindful eating is a powerful tool for developing a healthy relationship with food—physically, emotionally, and spiritually. It's about being fully present while eating, paying attention to hunger and fullness cues, and making intentional food choices. When we eat mindfully, we break free from emotional eating, stress eating, or mindless snacking that stems from boredom, habit, or negative emotions. Instead of turning to food for comfort, distraction, or reward, we learn to savor each bite, appreciate the nourishment food provides, and listen to our bodies with wisdom and self-discipline.

This practice isn't just about eating slower—it's about cultivating gratitude, self-discipline, and awareness. Food is a gift from God to sustain and strengthen our bodies, which are temples of the Holy Spirit. Mindfulness helps us shift our dependence away from food for comfort and redirect it to God, who alone can truly satisfy.

How Mindfully Do You Eat?

Take a moment to reflect on your eating habits by answering the following questions:

- Do you pay attention to when, why, and how you eat, or do you find yourself eating out of habit, convenience, or emotion?
- Are you aware of how different foods affect your mood, energy, and digestion?
- Do you fully taste and enjoy each bite, or do you eat quickly and distractedly?
- Do you stop eating when you're full, even if it's a food you love?
- Can you resist extra servings because you're satisfied, rather than because the food tastes good?

- Can you differentiate between true hunger and eating due to boredom, stress, or habit?
- Do you eat because you're hungry, or simply because it's mealtime?
- Are you typically able to eat just the right amount—not too little, not too much?

Take a moment to review your answers.

How many did you answer "no" to?

Which of these questions resonates most with you?

Which answer would you most like to change?

Now, envision yourself with your ideal relationship with food.

What does that look like for you?

What actions or thoughts would be different than they are now?

Your Mindful Eating Action Plan

1. Identify one or two food-related habits you want to change. Describe the habit in detail.

What is the habit?

What triggers the habit?

Does the habit occur at specific times or in specific situations?

2. Why do you want to change this habit?

3. How do you think you will feel once you make this change?

4. What is one positive step you can take today to diminish this habit?

Hunger is not always a response to a true physical need for nourishment. Often, we eat for reasons unrelated to providing our bodies with necessary nourishment, which can lead to unhealthy patterns and a disconnect from our natural hunger cues. Emotional eating, cravings, and mindless snacking can take a toll on both our physical health and our relationship with food. When we eat out of stress, sadness, boredom, or habit rather than true hunger, we may find ourselves consuming foods that do not nourish us, eating beyond fullness, or developing an unhealthy reliance on food for comfort. Becoming aware of why we eat is a crucial first step in making intentional, mindful choices that support our health and honor God. Consider the different types of hunger and how they may be influencing your eating habits:

- **Physical Hunger** – Your body's true need for nourishment.
- **Cravings** – A strong desire for a specific taste or texture, often unrelated to hunger.
- **Emotional Eating** – Eating in response to stress, sadness, anxiety, or as a reward.
- **Boredom Eating** – Eating to fill time, distract from responsibilities, or avoid discomfort.

Ask yourself:

Do I consistently eat to fuel my body with nourishing foods?

How often do I eat simply for pleasure or to satisfy cravings rather than hunger?

Do I use food as a way to relax, de-stress, or cope with emotions?

Do I find myself eating out of boredom or procrastination?

By becoming more aware of why you eat and making small, intentional changes, you can develop a healthier, more mindful relationship with food. Over time, practicing mindfulness in eating will help you tune into your body's natural cues and create sustainable habits that honor your temple—your body—as God intended.

Becoming aware of your eating habits is the first step in making lasting change. Over the next two weeks, we will take a Christ-centered approach to building habits that promote health and honor God.

Week 1

Choosing What is Beneficial

Day 1: Get The Full Life in Christ

Read: John 10:7-10

"God created it. Jesus died for it. The Spirit lives in it. I'd better take care of it."
– Pastor Rick Warren

Satan's mission is clear: he comes to steal, kill, and destroy. He wants to distract you from God's truth, keeping you from living in the full measure of His strength. He doesn't want you to become the best version of yourself—the person God created you to be. Satan tries to take the truth from you—the truth that you are a new creation, made beautiful in God's image, and that through Christ's strength, you can do all things. You were bought with a high price, and your life is now called to glorify God through discipleship.

Satan will often use seemingly harmless things—technology, social media, food, wine, or comfort—to distract you. He may not tempt you with obvious sins; instead, he subtly pulls you away from God, replacing Him as your source of comfort and joy.

What distractions might Satan be using in your life right now?

Imagine living the full life that Jesus promises in John 10:10.

What does that look like for you in:

Your relationship with God?

Your relationships with others?

Your self-esteem and how you view yourself?

Your relationship with food and how you care for yourself?

What's keeping you from living your life to the fullest?

For many, food becomes one of Satan's primary tools to steal joy and keep us from living in the fullness of who we are in Christ—walking in the power, wisdom, and self-discipline we've been given as new creations. Does this resonate with you?

- Do consuming thoughts about food steal your peace?
- Is food or drink a temptation in your life?
- Do you feel guilt or shame regarding your choices with food or overindulgence?
- Is your health compromised by consuming foods that negatively affect your body?

Our eating becomes harmful when it sabotages our health, undermines our confidence, or stirs up negative emotions like guilt and shame. It becomes sinful when it keeps us in bondage and robs us of the victory we are meant to live in, for our Lord and Savior came to break the chains of sin and lead us into lives of freedom and triumph.

Read: Galatians 5:13-25

We are equipped with God's Spirit, a gift given to us when we accept Jesus as our personal Savior. As we walk with the Lord, the Spirit is produced in our lives, and through God's strength, it is worked out in us so that we can fulfill His good purposes. The Spirit empowers us to align our will with the Lord's will. One of the Fruits of the Spirit is self-control, which can be defined, rather obviously, as 'the ability to control oneself.' From a Biblical perspective, it is better understood as 'controlling the power of the will under the operation of the Spirit.'

In contrast, the world tells us that self-control is something we must develop on our own, relying solely on our inner strength. While God has given us the ability to make choices, as Christians, we have something even greater—the power of the Holy Spirit. True self-control is not just a matter of willpower; it is something we cultivate through the guidance and strength of the Spirit. As we pursue His strength and learn to depend on the Spirit, we begin to live from a place of wisdom and intention rather than emotion. We learn to walk in step with the Holy Spirit, becoming people whose lives are marked by wisdom, self-discipline, and love—love for God, for others, and for ourselves. In every area, including how we think, make choices, build habits, and care for our bodies, we reflect more of who He is.

Think about a time when you relied solely on your willpower to change a habit or behavior. How did it turn out? How did it make you feel afterward?

In Ephesians 5:18, Paul contrasts being drunk on wine with being filled with the Spirit. In what situations do you struggle most with self-control or overconsumption?

The best antidote is to be filled with the Spirit. Remind yourself often: this journey is not just about weight loss, vanity, or conforming to the world's definition of appearance and attractiveness. It is a lifelong walk with Jesus, learning the fine art of self-discipline. A person who is filled with the Spirit is under His control and has divine help in gaining mastery over their own weaknesses. Paul explains this in Romans.

Read: Romans 8:5-9

Do you believe your relationship with food and physical health is part of a spiritual battle? Why or why not?

You belong to Christ, and the mighty Spirit of God lives in you. You can do all things through Christ, who gives you strength

(Philippians 4:13). Reflect on areas in your life where you need to grow in self-control. Lift these up to God right now, asking for His strength and presence. As you encounter challenges this week, pause in those moments and ask God once again to help you live in a way that honors Him.

Day 2: Choosing Life and Wisdom

One of Satan's most subtle yet powerful weapons is food. The very first temptation recorded in history was a food temptation—Eve eating the forbidden fruit in the Garden of Eden. The first temptation of Christ was also a food temptation—Satan urging Him to turn stones into bread after fasting for 40 days.

Esau, in a moment of hunger and impulsivity, sold his birthright for a bowl of stew, trading his inheritance and role in God's covenant for temporary satisfaction.

After being miraculously freed from slavery, the Israelites complained about missing the foods of Egypt, and their cravings made them long for bondage rather than trust in God's provision.

In 1 Corinthians, Paul rebuked some believers for dishonoring the sacredness of the Lord's Supper. While some overindulged in food and drink, turning a holy moment into selfish indulgence, others were left hungry.

It's no wonder the Bible commands us in 1 Corinthians 10:31, "Whether you eat or drink, or whatever you do, do everything for the glory of God." Satan uses food as a weapon to diminish our self-control, distort our priorities, and keep us from living out God's best. But God calls us to approach food with gratitude, wisdom, and self discipline.

"Do you not know that your bodies are temples of the Holy Spirit, who is in you, whom you have received from God? You are not your own; you were bought at a price. Therefore honor God with your bodies." - 1 Corinthians 6:19-20

Our bodies are temples of the Holy Spirit, and we are to honor God with them. When we choose to eat wisely—fueling our bodies with God-given foods and exercising self-control—eating becomes more than just a physical necessity. It becomes an act of faith, a way to treat our bodies as the sacred vessels He designed them to be.

Read: Ephesians 1:17-20

Hear Paul's prayer spoken over you: *I pray that you may have a spirit of wisdom that, in all areas of your life, you may know Him better.*

Can you think of any ways in which having a spirit of wisdom regarding your health, fitness, and physical well-being might help you to know God better?

Can you think of any benefits this might have for you as a disciple and follower of Christ?

"Today I have given you the choice between life and death, between blessings and curses. Now I call on heaven and earth to witness the choice you make. Oh, that you would choose life, so that you and your descendants might live!"
—Deuteronomy 30:19

God wants you to choose life. God wants you to choose blessings. God wants you to make wise choices. But to be wise about our choices, we must recognize that many of our actions, behaviors, and choices are governed by our habits. Our habits shape our lives. Unfortunately, even when we are aware of bad habits, it is difficult to replace them. It's one thing to *know* a habit is harmful; it's another thing to actually transform that habit into a beneficial one.

Why is this? Why is it so hard to replace habits that we *know* are harmful or, at the very least, aren't helping us grow, improve, and live exceptional lives?

First, you have most likely had these habits for a long time, and they've become comfortable. Habits don't form overnight, and many are deeply rooted in emotional needs. Some habits form out of fear, anxiety, or depression—perhaps in an attempt to fill a void or provide a sense of security.

Next, you may now *identify* with your habits. Someone might say, "I'm always late," "I worry by nature," or "I just don't have self-control" to explain their behavior. It's easy to confuse habits with identity, allowing them to define us. But your bad habits are *not* who you are! They are weaknesses, and they can be changed.

Do you believe your bad habits can be changed? Why or why not?

Bad habits are also hard to break because they offer immediate gratification. Learning to pursue *delayed* gratification—choosing a healthy, vibrant body in the future over the fleeting pleasure of eating for comfort or convenience—is difficult but possible.

"Where there is no revelation, people cast off restraint; but blessed is the one who heeds wisdom's instruction." - Proverbs 29:18

We strive to be Christians who demonstrate restraint and walk in wisdom in all areas of life, including our physical well-being. God provides the power to make healthy choices, exercise self-control, and live wisely.

"For God is working in you, giving you the desire and the power to do what pleases Him." —Philippians 2:13

God has a part—and you have a part—in both your spiritual and physical growth. He is working in you, giving you the desire and the power to do what is good, wise, and beneficial. But your role matters too.

Are you holding up your end of the bargain?

- How can you grow spiritually and take an active role in your faith?

- How can you be more intentional in caring for your physical health and well-being?

Everyone wants to be healthy, fit, strong, and confident—but only those who intentionally choose a healthy lifestyle will achieve it. Health and strength don't happen by accident. They require a decision. A commitment. A daily choice.

It's a lifetime of small, intentional choices that begin with the commitment to becoming the healthiest, strongest, and most vibrant version of yourself.

Each healthy choice you make shapes you. Compromise after compromise leads to defeat, but every small, wise decision builds a foundation for lifelong health and victory. Think of your choices as building blocks—each one stacked upon the next, forming something new. Slowly and steadily, your daily decisions will transform you into the person God is calling you to be.

Close your time in prayer, thanking God for the ability to make choices that align with His wisdom and design. Ask Him to reveal any habits or behaviors that are holding you back and to strengthen your self-discipline. Invite Him into your daily decisions regarding food, health, and fitness.

Take a moment to commit one specific action today that reflects the life and wisdom God calls you to walk in. What choice will you make today to honor Him with your body?

Day 3: Stewardship of the Body

Read: Matthew 25:14-30

Each of us has been given the gift of our earthly bodies, and our Heavenly Father wants us to care for this gift and manage it well. Just as Jesus teaches in the Parable of the Talents, He wants us to use everything He has given us to glorify Him. He calls us to invest in what we've been given, to use wisdom and discernment in how we handle our gifts. Ultimately, we desire to be faithful stewards and hear His loving words:

"Well done, good and faithful servant! You have been faithful with a few things; I will put you in charge of many things. Come and share your master's happiness!"

It's not about size; it's about stewardship—maximizing the gift of our bodies that God has given us. When we view exercise and healthy eating through this lens, it shifts our perspective. It's not about vanity or conforming to the world's standards of beauty; it's about taking care of the amazing gift God has graciously given. We know we will be held accountable for how we've used His gifts. Did we care for them and help them flourish, or did we neglect them? You have the opportunity to make exercise and healthy eating a form of praise and thanksgiving when you do it for the Lord.

How does your view of healthy eating, exercise, and caring for your physical health change when you shift your focus from losing weight or looking better to being a good steward of your body?

How can having a strong, healthy, and fit body be an investment in your walk with God and your life as a Christian?

In what ways might greater energy, a stronger body, and increased overall well-being help you live out the Fruit of the Spirit (love, joy, peace, patience, kindness, goodness, faithfulness, gentleness, and self-control)? For example, could you demonstrate more patience when you're not feeling tired or lethargic? Might practicing self-control with your eating habits help you develop greater self-control in your words and actions? Could you experience more joy when you are more energetic and confident in your body? How might improvements in your physical well-being contribute to your spiritual growth?

To be good stewards of our health and to maximize the gift of our bodies, we must conquer limiting beliefs. Satan wants to steal your joy and destroy your opportunity to live your life to the fullest. He wants to fill your mind with lies, which are often subtle and seemingly inconsequential. He may use food or alcohol as a temptation for comfort, or as a way to damage your confidence and leave you feeling powerless.

To defeat these lies, we must combat them with spiritual truths. Here are some examples of lies Satan may try to feed you:

- "I'm a failure; I'll never reach my goals."
- "This is too hard; I give up."
- "I deserve to indulge because I had a hard day."
- "I can eat whatever I want; it doesn't matter."
- "I hate my body."
- "I'm just meant to be this way."
- "This temptation is too strong; I might as well give in."

"We demolish arguments and every pretension that sets itself up against the knowledge of God, and we take captive every thought to make it obedient to Christ."

- 2 Corinthians 10:5

The battle begins in our minds. Lies and half-truths have no place in the mind of a Christian devoted to growing in the Lord. The only way to fight the lies the enemy tells us—about our bodies, health, or self-worth—is to take every thought captive and make it obedient to Christ. Changing our thoughts will change our behaviors, and the more we fill our minds with God's Word, the more we will grow in His likeness and live out His truth through the power of the Holy Spirit within us.

Steps to Overcome Limiting Beliefs

Assess Your Thoughts
Each day, evaluate your thoughts for limiting beliefs, half-truths, or lies. Ask yourself: *Does this thought align with Scripture? Is it true? Is it beneficial?* If not, take it captive—write it down if needed—and dismiss it. Set it aside. Refuse to let it take root in your mind.

Dismiss the Lies
Satan thrives on deception. If you don't actively combat false beliefs, they will shape your choices and habits and pull you away from the person God is calling you to become. Pay attention to the messages you tell yourself and reject anything that contradicts God's truth.

Replace Lies with Spiritual Truth
Don't stop at recognizing and removing lies—replace them with God's Word. Scripture is your most powerful weapon, and when you fill your mind with truth, it transforms both your thoughts and actions.

"It is the same with my word. I send it out, and it always produces fruit. It will accomplish all I want it to, and it will prosper everywhere I send it."
—Isaiah 55:11

God's Word will accomplish its purpose. As you meditate on Scripture, the Holy Spirit will renew your mind, reshape your behaviors, and lead you into greater wisdom, strength, and self-discipline. As you continue to practice replacing lies and half-truths with God's truth, you'll begin to recognize that you no longer have to rely on your own strength. Each choice, action, and habit becomes an opportunity for God's power to work in and through you. In this Spirit-led life, the Fruit of the Spirit—love, joy, peace, patience, kindness, goodness, faithfulness, gentleness, and self-control—will flourish more fully within you.

What are one or two lies or limiting beliefs you find yourself struggling with time and time again? What are they?

How can you replace these lies with truths from God's Word?

We are told in Scripture that the Kingdom of God is righteousness, peace, and joy in the Holy Spirit. If your thoughts or behaviors diminish your peace, joy, or your ability to walk in step with the Spirit, they are a concern to God. These thoughts hinder your ability to fulfill your purpose and keep you from becoming the best version of the person God created you to be.

Our minds are powerful, and our thoughts shape who we are and who we become. To live well and maximize our potential, we must be aware of—and take control of—our thoughts.

Here are a few Scriptures that highlight the importance of guarding our minds:

Week 1 | Choosing What is Beneficial

"Be careful what you think, because your thoughts run your life." - *Proverbs 4:23*

"Whatever is true, whatever is noble, whatever is right, whatever is pure, whatever is lovely, whatever is admirable—if anything is excellent or praiseworthy—think about such things."

Philippians 4:8

"For the Spirit God gave us does not make us timid, but gives us power, love, and self-discipline."

2 Timothy 1:7

"We take captive every thought to make it obedient to Christ."

2 Corinthians 10:5

In the week ahead, pay attention to your thought life. Take captive any thoughts that diminish your peace, joy, or health, and align them with the truth of God's Word. The battle begins in your mind—fight it wisely!

Day 4: Personal Willpower Alone Is Not Enough

Read: Galatians 5:16-18

We need willpower and discipline to create healthy habits, to grow in spiritual maturity, and to reflect Christ in all aspects of our lives. However, willpower and discipline alone can only take us so far. When we get weary, our mind, will, and emotions often push us toward what's easy—even if it's not what's best for us. But the Holy Spirit of God will guide us toward what strengthens us, helps us grow, and shapes us to become more like Him. He leads us into peace, joy, and the full life He desires for us. The key is staying open to His prompting and willing to follow His lead, especially in the small, everyday choices that shape who we're becoming.

Reflect on the past 24 to 48 hours. In what ways has God offered you escapes from temptation and strength through the Holy Spirit? Did you follow His lead, or did you choose your own way?

What were the results or consequences of your actions?

How can you learn from these experiences and rely more fully on the Holy Spirit in the future?

Satan, the father of lies, will do everything in his power to keep you from following the Holy Spirit's lead. He will tempt you with poor choices that pull you away from becoming your personal best in

God. He doesn't want you to rely on God's strength or grow in the Fruit of the Spirit. His lies are not innocent or harmless; they are intended to destroy your peace, joy, and fullness of life.

Perhaps you've already experienced the consequences of believing Satan's lies about food. Maybe you've faced health issues because of your food choices. Perhaps you've experienced shame, guilt, or hopelessness about changing your health or body.

What consequences have you faced from believing Satan's lies regarding food?

"You will know the truth, and the truth will set you free."
– John 8:32

As we grow in our walk with God, His words will dwell in our hearts, and the truth of His Word will set us free from Satan's lies.

Here are some common lies that we tend to believe about food, health, and physical well-being. Take time to reflect on which lies you may be susceptible to, and internalize God's truth to combat those lies.

Lies and Limiting Beliefs	**God's Truth**
"I deserve to indulge."	Food will not bring happiness—only the Lord will truly satisfy.
"I'm feeling down, I just want to sit down with a bag of chips."	*"Jesus answered, 'It is written: Man shall not live on bread alone, but on every word that comes from the mouth of God.'"* – Matthew 4:4
"It's been a hard day, I deserve ice cream to feel better.	*"Satisfy us in the morning with your unfailing love, that we may sing for joy and be glad all our days."* – Psalm 90:14
"I've tried everything. It's too hard. I give up."	*"So let's not get tired of doing what is good. At just the right time we will reap a harvest of blessing if we don't give up."* – Galatians 6:9

"I guess this is just who I am. Why bother?"

"I am sure that God, who began the good work in you, will keep on working in you until the day Jesus Christ comes again."

– Philippians 1:6

"I may as well quit. I'll never make a change."

We are not quitters. We are running a race that we will finish with strength.

"I can do all things through Christ who strengthens me."

– Philippians 4:13

"This is taking too long. Why bother?"

"Let us run with endurance the race that is set before us, looking unto Jesus, the author and finisher of our faith."

– Hebrews 12:1-2

"I hate my body." "I'm disgusting."	You are God's temple. The Bible describes temples as beautiful, magnificent, glorious, and wonderful. This is how the Heavenly Father sees you—and it's time for you to see yourself this way.
"I can't stand looking at myself."	*"I praise you because I am fearfully and wonderfully made; your works are wonderful, I know that full well."* – Psalm 139:14
"This is how I've always been. Nothing will ever change."	*"Don't you know that you yourselves are God's temple and that God's Spirit dwells in your midst?"* – 1 Corinthians 3:16
"I guess I'm just not the kind of person who can change."	*"If anyone belongs to Christ, he is a new person. The old life is gone. New life has begun."* – 2 Corinthians 5:17

"I'm just meant to stay this way."	You are a new creation in Christ. Past failures don't matter. Bring the Lord into this journey, and He will strengthen and guide you.

With which of these lies do you most likely struggle?

How has believing this lie affected you?

How can you remind yourself to replace these lies with the truth of God's Word?

Close your time in prayer, asking the Holy Spirit to guide your thoughts, choices, and actions. Reflect on areas where you've been relying on your own willpower instead of His strength. Ask God to reveal any lies you've been believing about yourself, your health, or your habits, and pray for wisdom to replace those lies with His truth. Commit to relying on the Spirit's power to help you grow in self-control and to make choices that honor Him. What is God calling you to surrender today so that you can walk in freedom and victory? Lift it up to Him now.

Day 5: Mastered by Nothing

"I have the right to do anything," you say—but not everything is beneficial. "I have the right to do anything"—but I will not be mastered by anything."
– 1 Corinthians 6:12

Take a moment to memorize this verse. Write it here, filling in the blanks:

"I have the right to do anything," you say—but not everything ________________. "I have the right to do anything"—but I will not be ____________________________."

This journey isn't about vanity; it's about self-control and discipline. But when a lack of control starts to define us, there's a problem. Do you rely on food for comfort more than you rely on God? When you are stressed, sad, or weary—or even when you are happy—do you turn to food instead of turning to God?

Do you feel capable of consistently making wise and beneficial choices when it comes to the food you eat?

Are there times when you feel you lack control in your food choices?

Do you ever feel mastered by food or cravings?

It doesn't matter if your weakness is ice cream, organic cookies, coffee, diet soda, or alcohol. If you are controlled by food, you are not controlled by the Holy Spirit.

As Christians, we are called to be in control of the choices we make, including those regarding what we put into our bodies. Every choice—big or small—reveals our character and shapes it over time. To grow in self-discipline, we must practice self-discipline. Like a muscle, it develops the more we use it.

In the week ahead, approach each food choice with this question: *"I have the right to eat this, but is it beneficial?"*

Do you think some of your food choices might change if you consistently asked yourself this question?

How do we consistently make wise and beneficial choices? How do we avoid being mastered by cravings? We pray. We ask for wisdom. Even in our health and food choices, we pray continually:

"Lord God, help me to choose the foods that will give me a strong, healthy, and capable body, ready to be used by You. Help me to experience the fruit of self-control given to me by the Holy Spirit."

God wants you to have wisdom in every area of your life, and He wants you to ask for it. Use every moment of craving and temptation as an opportunity to pray.

Read: James 1:2-5

Focus on verse 5:
"If any of you lacks wisdom, you should ask God, who gives generously to all without finding fault, and it will be given to you."

Every time you're tempted to overeat, eat the wrong foods, or eat for the wrong reasons, view it as an opportunity: an opportunity to pray, to lean into God's strength, and to grow in wisdom and self-discipline. When it comes to the healthy, abundant life God desires for you, you can't afford to continually compromise. Every small choice you make with prayer and wisdom strengthens not just your body but your character as a strong Christian. By approaching your health, fitness, and eating habits from a place of prayer, you begin to define yourself by your obedience to God—not by the numbers on a scale.

Even with this perspective, there will still be moments of struggle and failure. Paul understood this struggle when he said:

"I want to do what is good, but I don't. I don't want to do what is wrong, but I do it anyway."

Romans 7:19

This is such a relatable statement! Haven't we all felt this way? Take some time to read the full passage:

Read: Romans 7:14-25

The truths in this passage can feel overwhelming—Paul points out the painful reality of our sinful nature and how it prevents us from living the lives we desire. But Paul doesn't highlight our weakness to discourage us. Instead, he is preparing us for the joy of God's gracious provision, which is described in Romans 8. By acknowledging the struggle in Romans 7, we are better equipped to receive the encouragement that follows.

Read: Romans 8:9-17

What does it mean to you that the same Spirit who raised Jesus from the dead lives in you? How can this truth empower you to overcome weaknesses and live in greater alignment with God's will?

Close your time in prayer, asking God to help you identify anything in your life—whether food, habits, or cravings—that may be mastering you. Surrender those areas to Him, and ask for the wisdom and self-control to make choices that are beneficial and honor Him. Reflect on how you can rely on God's strength, rather than your own, to overcome temptations. Commit to approaching every decision this week with the question: "Is this beneficial?" Trust that, through prayer and the Holy Spirit, you can live a life that reflects His glory.

Week 2

Living by the Spirit

Day 1: A Soul at Rest

Read: 1 Corinthians 9:24-27

In *Soul Keeping*, John Ortberg writes, "When my will is consistently, freely, joyfully aligned with what I most deeply value, my soul finds rest." When your choices, thoughts, and actions are in harmony with your deepest values, you experience wholeness. But when you live with half-hearted devotion—wanting one thing but doing another—your soul becomes strained and divided.

God designed us for harmony: our will directing our mind, and our mind directing our body. When we live in this alignment, surrendered to Him, our soul is at rest. But when we live divided lives, we experience inner turmoil—a life where our actions don't match our beliefs or good intentions.

Think of a person who desires financial freedom but keeps making impulsive purchases. Or someone who wants to honor their health but turns to chips or ice cream for comfort. It's like pressing the accelerator and brake at the same time—going nowhere and wearing yourself down in the process.

In what areas of your life are your actions not aligned with your beliefs, goals or desires for your future?

What is the "good" you want to do but find difficult to act on?

What habits, thoughts, or behaviors might be dividing your soul?

Parker Palmer once wrote, "The divided life is a wounded life, and the soul keeps calling us to heal the wound." Healing this division begins with surrendering your will to God. When your will is fully submitted to Him, your mind can take control over your thoughts, and your body can act in alignment with those thoughts.

However, the real danger lies in the small habits, thoughts, and actions that don't align with our deepest goals or vision for our lives—yet over time, they become comfortable and normalized. We dismiss unhealthy patterns, justifying them because they meet a need in the moment. But to live with purpose, we must learn to make choices based on vision, not fleeting emotions. Otherwise, harmful behaviors—like turning to food for comfort, staying trapped in cycles of debt, or filling our days with meaningless distractions—start to feel acceptable and even normal. Character is the ability to follow through on a decision after the emotion of making that decision is gone.

What habitual thoughts, feelings, or actions might you be accepting as normal, even though they hinder your growth or keep you from your deepest goals?

How might surrendering these to God bring your soul into alignment and rest?

How can submitting your health and fitness goals to God create harmony in other areas of your life?

Listen to this very familiar passage from the book of Romans, *The Message* version:

"If the power of sin within me keeps sabotaging my best intentions, I obviously need help! I realize that I don't have what it takes. I can will it, but I can't do it. I decide to do good, but I don't really do it; I decide not to do bad, but then I do it anyway. My decisions, such as they are, don't result in actions. Something has gone wrong deep within me and gets the better of me every time. It happens so regularly that it's predictable. The moment I decide to do good, sin is there to trip me up." - Romans 7:18-21

This passage reflects the struggle we all face—the tension between our desires and our actions, between what we know is right and what we actually do. Yet, the solution is clear: Jesus Christ. Through His Spirit, we are given the power, love, and self-discipline to align our lives with God's design.

God's design for our health is that we nourish our bodies with the foods He created, that we move and strengthen them, and that we live with energy, diligence, and purpose. He calls us to be industrious, hard-working, and vibrant, caring for the bodies He has entrusted to us. Our bodies are not our own; they are temples of the Holy Spirit. When we offer our bodies and all that they are capable of to God, we engage in a profound act of worship, as Paul reminds us in Romans 12:1:

"Therefore, I urge you, brothers and sisters, in view of God's mercy, to offer your bodies as a living sacrifice, holy and pleasing to God—this is your true and proper worship."

Caring for our physical well-being isn't just about health—it's about honoring God with our lives, using our strength and energy to serve Him fully, and living in alignment with His purpose for us.

Every day, we are becoming someone. Every choice, every habit, every thought shapes us into the person we are becoming. Are you growing in the Fruit of the Spirit—love, joy, peace, patience, kindness, goodness, faithfulness, gentleness, and self-control—or are you being mastered by something else? It's a process, a lifetime of learning to submit our will to God and live in harmony with His purposes.

Close your time in prayer, asking God to reveal any areas of division in your life where your thoughts, desires, or actions don't align with His will. Ask Him for the wisdom to recognize these patterns and the strength to surrender them to Him. Pray for a soul at rest, fully aligned with God's purposes, and for the power, love, and self-discipline to take steps each day toward the person He is calling you to become.

Day 2: Honoring God with Your Entire Life

"Therefore, I urge you, brothers and sisters, in view of God's mercy, to offer your bodies as a living sacrifice, holy and pleasing to God—this is your true and proper worship. Do not conform to the pattern of this world, but be transformed by the renewing of your mind. Then you will be able to test and approve what God's will is—his good, pleasing and perfect will."

Romans 12:1-2

God wants you to live an exceptional life. He desires to use you in extraordinary ways and for you to experience the full, abundant life He's planned for you. Yet many Christians never fully embrace the power they have in Christ or the presence of the Holy Spirit in their daily lives. Perhaps today is your invitation to begin walking in that power, one faithful step at a time.

We find peace, joy, and satisfaction—living our best, most Christ-centered lives—when we grow in the Fruit of the Spirit. These virtues (love, joy, peace, patience, kindness, goodness, faithfulness, gentleness, and self-control) are not just behaviors we adopt to be "better" Christians. They are blessings that transform our lives.

In today's culture, the idea of viewing our bodies as "living sacrifices" is countercultural. Romans 12:1 challenges us to see our bodies not as objects for self-serving purposes or possessions we own, but as vessels meant to bring glory to God. The world often tells us something very different. Many see the body as a personal project—something to sculpt, perfect, or display in pursuit of unrealistic and superficial standards of beauty, often rooted in sex appeal rather than substance or worth. Others treat the body as something of little value—believing only the spiritual life matters, and that how they care for their physical body has no real connection to their character, witness, or effectiveness as an ambassador for Christ. But Scripture reminds us that our bodies are not our own; they are gifts from God, temples of the Holy Spirit (1 Corinthians 6:19-20). When we offer our daily lives and physical bodies to the Lord, it becomes a true act of worship.

When we offer our bodies as living sacrifices, we declare: "Lord, use me fully—my mind, my strength, my energy, my hands and my feet, and all that I am capable of—for Your glory." This mindset shifts our focus. Instead of striving for external validation or feeling shame for not "measuring up," we begin to steward our bodies with purpose, gratitude, and intentionality. It's no longer about how we look, the number on the scale, or how we compare to others. It's about how well we are stewarding our mental, physical, and emotional health as an act of worship. This is the true worship Paul describes.

How does viewing your body as a "living sacrifice" change your perspective on health and fitness?

In what ways does your physical health impact your ability to serve God and others?

Are there habits or thought patterns preventing you from fully offering your body as a sacrifice to God?

True transformation starts with a renewed mindset. Shift your focus from outward goals like losing weight or looking better to a spiritual perspective. Ask God to renew your mind regarding your health and fitness. Pray for wisdom to understand how caring for your physical body impacts your mood, energy, and relationships.

"God, help me to demonstrate wisdom and grow in the fruit of self-discipline in this area of my life. Help me to understand how honoring my body as a living sacrifice impacts every part of my life. Align my health goals with Your will, and help me steward this gift well."

"For this reason I remind you to fan into flame the gift of God, which is in you through the laying on of my hands. For the Spirit God gave us does not make us timid, but gives us power, love and self-discipline."

2 Timothy 1:6-7

Every day, in every aspect of your life—including your physical health—seek God's will and wisdom. He desires for you to live a full, blessed, and abundant life, and to bless others through your obedience and discipline. Paul's charge to "fan into flame the gift of God" is a reminder that the gifts He's placed within us—like self-discipline—are not passive. They are meant to be stirred, strengthened, and grown. Every time you make a healthy choice, every time you show restraint, say no to temptation, or act in wisdom rather than impulse, you're fanning into flame the gift of the Holy Spirit. Picture that gift like a glowing ember—something God has placed within you, but which requires your active participation to grow. Don't let it remain small and dormant. Fan it, tend to it, and watch it grow into a powerful flame that shapes every part of your life—your habits, your thoughts, your health, and your journey toward becoming your best for God's glory.

We are called to be radically intentional in every area of our lives, including health. The devil wants to keep us in "default mode," living passively and stuck in easy, comfortable habits. But God calls us to rise above that. Jesus wants us to strive for excellence, to care for the bodies He has entrusted to us, and to live with purpose. Staying comfortable might feel easy, but it isn't God's best for you. You were made for more!

Don't just dream about what you can achieve in your health. Dream about what Jesus can do through your commitment, effort, and trust in Him.

Close your time in prayer, asking God to help you view your health as an act of worship and an offering to Him. Ask Him to renew your mind and strengthen your self-discipline. Pray for the courage to live with radical intentionality, stewarding your body to glorify Him and serve others. Surrender your goals and efforts to Him, trusting that He will work through you for His glory.

Day 3: The Fruit of Self-Discipline

Like a city whose walls are broken through is a person who lacks self-control."
Proverbs 25:28

Self-discipline is essential to living a life that honors God. Without it, we become vulnerable—like a city with broken walls, unprotected and easily overcome. In this state, we struggle with unhealthy habits, poor decisions, and spiritual stagnation. By building self-discipline in areas such as nutrition, exercise, and daily habits, we practice the skill of doing what we don't feel like doing, even when it's difficult or inconvenient. This practice shifts our focus from instant gratification to living for a greater purpose and long-term goals. Ultimately, self-discipline is vital not only for our health but also for our relationships, spiritual growth, and character development.

However, God has not left us to face these challenges alone. He has given us His Spirit, equipping us with the fruit of self-control.

"*But the Holy Spirit produces this kind of fruit in our lives: love, joy, peace, patience, kindness, goodness, faithfulness, gentleness, and self-control. There is no law against these things!*"

Galatians 5:22-23

Self-discipline is not just about willpower; it is a gift cultivated through the Holy Spirit. It allows us to align our lives with God's purposes, transforming our thoughts, habits, and actions to reflect His character. But cultivating this fruit requires intentional effort.

For many, finding the right meal plan or workout program isn't the real problem—lack of self-control is. Instead of focusing solely on external factors like losing weight or achieving a certain body image, shift your focus to building a spirit of self-discipline in this area of your life. When self-discipline is developed through the Spirit, it impacts every aspect of life—not just our health, but our ability to resist temptation, make wise decisions, and grow in faith.

Lack of self-discipline leaves us vulnerable, not only in our physical health but in our spiritual lives as well. Too many Christians fail to fully experience the power they have in Christ and the presence of the Holy Spirit in every aspect of their lives. The power of Christ is meant to transform our thoughts, words, actions, habits, relationships, and even the way we honor our bodies as temples of the Holy Spirit.

"For physical training is of some value, but godliness has value for all things, holding promise for both the present life and the life to come."

1 Timothy 4:8

Paul acknowledges that physical training holds value. While it isn't the most important thing, it still plays a role in our lives. Honoring our bodies through healthy habits offers both spiritual and physical benefits. Caring for our bodies is a practical and daily opportunity to grow in self-discipline. It's a tangible way to live out the verse: "I will not be mastered by anything" (1 Corinthians 6:12).

When our will and actions align with our goals and values, we experience wholeness. Unfortunately, this isn't always the case. Many people struggle with the tension between what they desire—to be healthy, strong, and disciplined—and what they actually do. Even with the best intentions, we often fall into patterns that contradict our long-term goals. But when we submit our will to God and live in harmony with His purposes, we begin to blossom into the person He designed us to be.

God designed us to live in perfect harmony, where our choices, thoughts, desires, and behaviors align with His design and intention. When we function as He intended, our wills are fully surrendered to Him, our minds are guided by that surrendered will, and our bodies follow in obedience to a mind that is under God's direction.

In this alignment, we act with wisdom and self-control, making decisions based on what is right and beneficial rather than on fleeting emotions or desires. This is how we find peace and live the vibrant, joyful lives Jesus came to give us (John 10:10).

Exercise and healthy eating are tools God has given us to enhance our lives, helping to manage stress, anxiety, and anger while building energy, stamina, and longevity. When we care for our bodies, we improve our mood and mental health, become better equipped to serve God and others, and experience greater joy and clarity in our daily lives. Satan, however, often uses health and fitness as a weapon against believers, attacking our self-control and distorting our views. Here are some ways he works:

Diminishing self-control: Using food, drink, or other comforts to weaken our discipline.

Damaging health: Reducing our energy, longevity, and mental well-being, which affects our ability to serve God effectively.

Bringing shame and guilt: Making us feel unworthy or defeated.

Distorting fitness: Turning it into a source of vanity, comparison, or self-loathing rather than stewardship and gratitude.

When we recognize these attacks, we can fight back with the power of the Holy Spirit, asking for wisdom and strength to honor God in all areas of our lives, including our health.

What would Jesus say about your health and fitness? Jesus likely wouldn't place an overemphasis on these things. He would remind us that our worth doesn't come from our physical bodies or how others perceive us. Yet, He would also encourage us to use what we've been given for His glory—living with wisdom and self-discipline.

Jesus might remind us to use food as a source of gratitude and sustenance rather than as a replacement for God's comfort. He would encourage us to strengthen our bodies and prioritize our health so that we can serve God and others with energy, joy, and vitality. He would call us to remove anything that hinders our growth in the Fruit of the Spirit, urging us to become our best for His glory.

Are there areas of your life where you are lacking self-discipline?

How might focusing on building self-discipline help you grow in your spiritual life?

What steps can you take today to align your actions and habits with the goals and values God has placed on your heart?

Close your time in prayer, asking God to strengthen your self-discipline through the power of His Spirit. Surrender any areas where you feel weak or vulnerable, and ask Him to help you align your thoughts, habits, and actions with His purposes. Commit to seeking Him daily as you strive to become the person He has called you to be, and trust in His power to transform your life for His glory.

Day 4: God's Blueprint for Health

"Then God said, 'I give you every seed-bearing plant on the face of the whole earth and every tree that has fruit with seed in it. They will be yours for food.'"
Genesis 1:29

"Everything that lives and moves about will be food for you. Just as I gave you the green plants, I now give you everything."

Genesis 9:3

"He has shown kindness by giving you rain from heaven and crops in their seasons; he provides you with plenty of food and fills your hearts with joy."
Acts 14:17

God's Word speaks clearly about His provision for us, especially when it comes to the food we eat. From the very beginning, He provided every seed-bearing plant and tree that bears fruit, filling the earth with plants and animals for our nourishment. In Acts 14:17, Paul reminds us of God's kindness, saying, "He provides you with plenty of food and fills your hearts with joy."

God designed both the earth and our bodies to work in perfect harmony. The natural, whole foods He created are not only meant to sustain us physically but also to bless us mentally, emotionally, and spiritually. Yet, in a culture filled with processed, convenient, and artificial choices, it's easy to drift away from God's blueprint. What would happen if we intentionally returned to the foods God originally provided and embraced His design for health?

When we nourish our bodies with whole, unprocessed foods as God intended, our minds become sharper, our emotions more stable, and our spirits more connected to Him. Proper nutrition fuels our brains, enhancing mental clarity so we can fully engage with God's Word, focus during prayer, and discern His guidance. It also strengthens emotional stability, allowing us to be more present, compassionate, and patient in our relationships. When we feel our best mentally and emotionally, we communicate with kindness, handle challenges with grace, and show up fully for those God has placed in our lives.

Beyond mental and emotional well-being, eating God-given foods has practical benefits that equip us to live with energy and endurance. A diet rich in whole, nourishing foods stabilizes mood, balances blood sugar levels, and reduces feelings of irritability, anxiety, and fatigue. Instead of feeling sluggish or drained, we are energized and strengthened to steward our time well—caring for our families, working in ministry, and pursuing our God-given callings with vitality.

A meaningful, yet often overlooked, benefit of honoring our health through proper nutrition is spiritual. Choosing the foods God created for us can become an act of worship, a way of saying, "Lord, I honor the body You've given me, and I trust Your design for my health." Preparing and eating whole foods can become a simple moment of gratitude—an intentional act of choosing what God designed to nourish us. Even in the small, daily choices we make about the foods we eat, we have an opportunity to honor Him by demonstrating wisdom and thanksgiving, following His blueprint for health, and stewarding our bodies well—fully embracing the gift of physical, mental, and emotional well-being that God-given foods provide.

Just as nourishing our bodies with the foods God intended is a way to honor Him, so is moving our bodies with purpose and care. Regular physical activity is one of the most effective ways we can care for the bodies God has given us. Exercise might not always be easy, but the benefits are undeniable. When you move your body regularly, you feel stronger, more energetic, and more capable of handling whatever the day brings. You build stamina for everything from chasing after your kids to serving others with energy and joy. It helps you think more clearly, sleep more soundly, and feel more balanced emotionally. Exercise is a powerful tool for managing stress, lifting your mood, and even easing anxiety.

It's not just about what it does for your body—exercise can clear your mind and reset your focus. It's a healthy escape from the noise of life—a space to clear your head, release stress, and let go of frustration, anxiety, or worry. You don't need to be perfect or follow a rigid routine; you simply need to show up, keep going, and remember that every bit of effort is an investment in your strength, your mindset, and your ability to live well for God's glory.

Practical Steps to Align Your Health with God's Design

Begin each day by praying, "Lord, how can I honor You with my body today?" Seek His wisdom in your choices about food, exercise, and self-care. Don't feel overwhelmed by trying to make drastic changes overnight. Instead, commit to one small change this week—like adding more vegetables to your meals, taking a short walk daily, or swapping processed snacks for whole foods. Small, consistent steps lead to big transformations. Shift your focus from viewing healthy habits as a burden to seeing them as a way to glorify God. When you choose to eat nourishing foods or exercise, remind yourself that you're doing it as an act of worship and stewardship.

Your health journey isn't just about looking better or losing weight—it's about equipping yourself to serve God's Kingdom with strength, energy, and joy. Keep your eyes fixed on Him, and trust that He will guide you every step of the way.

How might eating God-given foods improve not only your physical health but also your mental, emotional, and spiritual well-being?

What small step can you take today to align your eating and exercise habits with God's design?

How can you view nutrition and exercise as acts of worship and gratitude?

Close your time in prayer by thanking God for the resources and tools He has given you to care for your body, mind, and spirit. Ask Him to help you make choices that reflect His wisdom and plan for your health. If there are areas where you've struggled with self-discipline, surrender them to Him and invite Him to guide your steps. Commit to seeing food and exercise as ways to honor Him, and ask for His help in taking care of your body in a way that brings Him glory.

Day 5: The Problem is Not Lack of Self-Control

"Therefore, if anyone is in Christ, the new creation has come: The old has gone, the new is here!"

2 Corinthians 5:17

If food or eating in any way feels like a battle for you, the problem isn't that you lack self-control. You've already been given a spirit of power and self-discipline—you just need to learn how to live it out.

In Christ, you've been given a new heart and a new spirit, along with the power for real and lasting change. A vital part of this new heart is the willpower you receive as a new creation in Christ. Your will matters deeply in your Christian walk because it's your moment-by-moment choices that determine whether you're living according to God's Spirit—or simply reacting based on your own emotions, cravings, or impulses.

Philippians 2:13 reminds us, *"For God is the one who works in you to will and to act according to His good purpose."* God is not only shaping your desires—He's also giving you the power to act on them, leading you step by step toward the person He's shaping you to become.

It is our will—the ability to choose—and the power to carry it out that creates the pathway for God's love and strength to move from our hearts into our lives. Our bodies and actions become the conduit for His Spirit to flow. With every moment-by-moment decision, we are either opening that passageway—allowing His power to work through us—or closing it off, limiting the transformation He desires to bring. It's not just what we believe in our hearts, but what we choose to do with our minds and bodies that determines how fully we walk in His strength and purpose.

Loving God with all our heart not only means asking Him into our lives—at which point we receive His supernatural presence and power—but also allowing His love, wisdom, and strength to become the motivation for everything we do.

Romans 8:5 says, *"Those who live according to the flesh set their minds on the things of the flesh, but those who live according to the Spirit set their minds on the things of the Spirit."* That verse draws a clear line between a life shaped by God and a life shaped by self.

It's important to understand that willpower has two distinct components. First, we have God's supernatural will and power, which was given to us when we accepted Christ as Savior. Through the Holy Spirit, He shows us what is right and gives us the strength to resist temptation and choose what honors Him. But we also have our own free will—the freedom to follow His lead or to follow our own thoughts, feelings, and desires.

So we constantly face a choice:

- Will we make faith-based choices, saying, *"Not as I will, but as You will,"* as Jesus did in Matthew 26:39?
- Or will we make emotion-based choices, following what feels good in the moment instead of what honors God, shapes our character, and helps us become more like Christ?

God's supernatural gift of self-discipline enables us to choose His ways over our cravings, emotions, and urges—and gives us the strength to carry them out. It's what we choose, moment by moment, that determines the direction of our lives.

When we live according to emotion, we don't lose the power of God that was given to us through Christ—but we can severely limit its impact in our lives. Through our continual choices, we either allow His power to shape us or we diminish its influence, leaving ourselves more vulnerable to temptation and the pull of sin. Every time we make emotional choices—choosing a self-guided path over a God-guided one—we hinder the work He desires to do in and through us.

This creates a double-minded life—one part surrendered to God, and another still driven by self. This kind of emotional response is frequently fueled by past hurts, hidden insecurities, or unmet needs. These are the things that keep us stuck, reacting emotionally instead of living intentionally.

What buried emotions might be influencing your choices more than you realize?

When we're controlled by emotion rather than being guided by the Holy Spirit, we're vulnerable to the enemy's influence. Satan seeks to manipulate our thoughts, stir our insecurities, and keep us focused on our hurts instead of God's promises. He wins when we fail to *"take every thought captive"* (2 Corinthians 10:5) and allow past wounds to drive our habits and actions.

But you are not a slave to the past—not to past hurts, not to past failures, not to previous insecurities or limiting beliefs.

"For we know that our old self was crucified with him so that the body ruled by sin might be done away with... anyone who has died has been set free from sin."
Romans 6:6–7

In Christ, you have everything you need to overcome. If you choose to obey and trust Him, His strength will carry you through every temptation, every moment of weakness, and every urge toward choices that don't reflect His best for you.

"I have been crucified with Christ. It is no longer I who live, but Christ who lives in me."

Galatians 2:20

Each day, in every choice, we have an opportunity to allow God's Spirit to move through us—to fill our minds, shape our habits, and guide our actions. This isn't a one-time decision. It's a moment-by-moment choice to be guided by His Spirit.

Think of your journey like driving at night. Your headlights don't light up the entire road—they only show you the next few feet. The same is true for your health journey. Don't get overwhelmed by the big picture. Focus on your next faithful step.

Ask yourself:

- What can I do today to care for my body?
- How can I demonstrate self-discipline in the next choice I have to make?

These small, intentional decisions begin to add up. Over time, they shape who you are becoming.

Transformation doesn't happen all at once.
It's the result of consistent, Spirit-led choices: choosing nourishing, God-given foods… choosing to exercise… choosing rest when needed… and choosing to keep your heart rooted in Christ. These are the things that strengthen your character, deepen your faith, and move you toward the life God desires for you.

God is with you in this. His Spirit strengthens your self-discipline, renews your mind, and empowers you to overcome.

Close your time in prayer. Thank God for the gifts of His Spirit that He has placed within you.
Ask Him to help you fan into flame the spirit of self-discipline and surrender the areas where you feel weak or stuck.
Invite Him to guide each decision you face today, and trust that with every small, faithful step, He is shaping you into the person He created you to be.

Bonus Leader Guide

Honoring My Temple

Leader Guide Introduction

WELCOME

Welcome to the *Honoring My Temple* Leader Guide. This guide is designed to help you facilitate meaningful discussions and foster deep connections within your small group as you journey through these devotionals. The content of this book is not just about food and health—it is about spiritual transformation, breaking free from distractions, and learning to honor God with our bodies, minds, and choices.

Satan's tactics are subtle, yet powerful. He uses food, comfort, and distractions to keep us from fully living in God's truth. But as we seek to align our habits with Christ's strength, we can walk in freedom, self-discipline, and purpose. These devotionals challenge us to recognize where we may be turning to food, habits, or unhealthy coping mechanisms instead of relying on God's sustaining power.

As you lead this small group, know that transformation happens in community. God designed us to encourage and uplift one another, to hold each other accountable, and to grow in faith together. This journey is not just about personal change—it's about creating a space where women can be honest, vulnerable, and empowered to walk in the fullness of God's plan for them. May this time together deepen your faith, strengthen your self-discipline, and draw you closer to the Lord and to one another.

Over the next three weeks, I pray that you and your small group will embrace every opportunity to grow stronger—physically, mentally, and spiritually. This guide is here to help you facilitate discussions, build deeper connections, and hold each other accountable as you pursue a healthier, more vibrant life in Christ.

Remember, God is calling you to grow, and He's also calling you to be a source of strength and encouragement for others on their journey. As you use this guide, trust that the Lord will work through you to bless and inspire those around you. Together, you will grow in wisdom, self-discipline, and physical and spiritual vitality.

I'm excited to begin this journey with you and look forward to seeing how God will move in your life and in the lives of those in your group. Let's get started!

Leading Your "Honoring My Temple" Small Group

As you begin the journey of leading a small group through *Honoring My Temple*, you have two options for structuring your discussions. You may choose to focus solely on the *Honoring My Temple* devotionals, or you can pair this Leader Guide with SoulStrength Fit's corresponding faith-based fitness program, *Honoring My Temple*, found in the SoulStrength Fit Faith-Based Fitness Program Library. www.soulstrengthfit.com

Regardless of your choice, this Leader Guide is designed to equip you with the tools necessary to facilitate meaningful discussions, foster deeper connections, and support others in their walk with the Lord.

Structure of This Leader Guide

This guide is designed to be used over three meetings:

1. **Meeting One:** Discuss the introduction. This session can take place before participants begin reading the book.
2. **Meeting Two:** Discuss reflections from Week 1 of the devotionals.
3. **Meeting Three:** Discuss reflections from Week 2 of the devotionals.

Each meeting will provide a structured framework to encourage reflection, personal insight, and group support. This approach emphasizes building a strong community, deepening relationships, and fostering spiritual growth through the teachings and scriptures explored in the daily devotionals.

Option 1: Using Honoring My Temple Alone

If your group is focusing exclusively on the *Honoring My Temple* devotionals, this Leader Guide provides a structured framework for a three-week small group study. Each session is thoughtfully designed to give members the opportunity to discuss the devotionals, share how the messages spoke to them personally, and discuss the ways God is working in their hearts. It's an opportunity to talk through key takeaways, personal convictions, and real-life applications. This small group study encourages meaningful connection, strengthens both faith and health journeys, and creates space for authentic conversations around what it looks like to honor God with our daily choices.

Option 2: Pairing with SoulStrength Fit's Honoring My Temple Faith-Based Fitness Program

For a comprehensive mind-body-spirit approach, consider pairing the *Honoring My Temple* devotionals with SoulStrength Fit's *Honoring My Temple Faith-Based Fitness Program.* This option gives your group the practical tools to apply the message of the devotionals to their daily lives. It includes corresponding strength-training workouts that incorporate prayer and ongoing Bible study and reflection, as well as Christ-centered nutrition coaching to help members develop healthy, sustainable eating habits. Together, this pairing supports lasting transformation—spiritually, mentally, and physically.

The program includes:

- Three weekly faith-based workouts that correspond with the daily devotionals.
- Comprehensive nutrition guidance and health coaching.
- Access to a full library of subsequent programs that feature ongoing devotionals and Christian workouts, ensuring continuous growth and support.

This Leader Guide provides you with all the tools needed to facilitate weekly meetings, offering your group the opportunity to come together for accountability, encouragement, and sustained growth in both their faith and fitness journeys. When you pair the *Honoring My Temple* devotionals with the Faith-Based Fitness Program, your group will build strength—both physically and spiritually—while putting faith into action through simple, meaningful habits. You can learn more and sign up at www.soulstrengthfit.com.

Getting Started

Whether your group chooses to focus just on the devotionals or add in the fitness and nutrition components, this Leader Guide is here to help you lead with confidence. Pick the option that works best for your group, and get ready to grow together—spiritually, physically, and in the everyday choices that honor God.

Tips for Leading Your Group

Creating a supportive and engaging small group environment is essential to the success of your meetings. Start by encouraging and supporting your group.

Foster group interaction by creating a welcoming and nurturing environment where members feel comfortable sharing their experiences, struggles, and victories. Ask questions with genuine interest and warmth while actively listening to individual responses. Remember, the process and the discussion are more valuable than arriving at specific answers.

As a leader, guide the conversation with flexibility. Feel free to reword the questions provided in the Leader Guide if needed, and decide when to spend more or less time on certain topics. You have the discretion to skip or add questions based on the needs of your group. Strive to prevent anyone, including yourself, from dominating the conversation, and gently redirect the discussion when necessary. Conversely, allow members to participate at their own comfort level. Not everyone needs to respond to every question, and it's okay if it takes time for some members to feel comfortable enough to share. Remember, your role is to guide the conversation, not carry it.

When questions arise within the group, do your best to provide answers. However, you don't need to have all the answers as a Small Group Leader. It's perfectly fine to say, "I'm not sure about that one, let me look into it." This moment can also be an opportunity to open the question up for group input and discussion, fostering a collaborative learning environment.

Your role as a leader is not to be an expert but to encourage and support your group as you all grow together in faith and health. Trust that God will work through your discussions, and let Him guide you as you lead others on this journey.

Session 1: Introduction & Mindful Eating

Welcome & Opening Prayer

Start the meeting by welcoming everyone and opening with prayer. Encourage members to pray for guidance, wisdom, and an open heart as they begin this journey together.

Introductions & Building Community

Encourage each member to introduce themselves. Here are some questions you may want to choose from to build community and foster connection:

- What brought you to this group, and what do you hope to gain from it?
- What is one thing you're passionate about outside of your faith?
- Do you have a favorite Bible verse or life verse?
- What's one area of your life where you're seeking to grow spiritually?

Mindful Eating Discussion

Mindful eating is about being fully present while eating, recognizing hunger and fullness cues, and making intentional food choices.

Ask: Which of these is most problematic for you? Use the following questions to help guide discussion:

• Do you feel in control of your food choices, or do you often feel like they're driven by habit or emotion?
• Do you use food as a way to relax, de-stress, or cope with emotions? How often do you eat simply for pleasure or to satisfy cravings rather than hunger?
• Do you find yourself eating out of boredom or procrastination?

After discussing, encourage group members to take it a step further and reflect on one or two food-related habits they want to improve. Creating a simple action plan can help bring clarity and accountability.

Use these prompts to guide the process:

• What is the habit you want to change?
• What typically triggers this habit? (Time of day, emotions, situations?)
• What is one positive step you can take today to start changing it?

Types of Hunger

Hunger is not always a response to a true physical need for nourishment. Often, we eat for reasons unrelated to providing our bodies with necessary nourishment, which can lead to unhealthy patterns and a disconnect from our natural hunger cues.

- **Physical Hunger** – Your body's true need for nourishment.
- **Cravings** – A strong desire for a specific taste or texture, often unrelated to hunger.
- **Emotional Eating** – Eating in response to stress, sadness, anxiety, or as a reward.
- **Boredom Eating** – Eating to fill time, distract from responsibilities, or avoid discomfort.

Ask:

- Which type of hunger do you struggle with most?
- When are you most likely to eat simply for pleasure, to satisfy cravings, or to use food as a way to relax, de-stress, or cope with emotions?
- How does your mindset around food change when you're tired, stressed, or overwhelmed?
- Have you ever invited God into your decision-making when it comes to food or eating habits? What would it look like to do that more often?

Closing Prayer & Prayer Requests

Invite each member to share a personal prayer request. This fosters openness and community. Encourage members to pray for self-discipline, wisdom, and strength to make mindful choices that honor God.

Encourage members to spend time reflecting on their mindful eating habits during the week and apply what they've discussed.

Looking Ahead

In the next session, members will discuss reflections from Week 1 of the devotionals. Encourage everyone to take notes on their experiences and any insights they gain from their mindful eating journey.

Session 2: Renewing Your Mind & Building Self-Discipline

Welcome & Opening Prayer

Begin by welcoming everyone and opening with prayer. Encourage members to pray for transformation and strength as they work toward aligning their health and fitness goals with God's plan.

Living Life to the Fullest

Read John 10:10

Ask: What does living life to the fullest look like for you in:

- Your relationship with God?
- Your relationships with others?

- Your self-esteem and how you view yourself?
- Your relationship with food and how you care for yourself?

What's keeping you from living your life to the fullest?

The Spiritual Battle in Health and Fitness

Read Romans 8:5-9

Ask:

- Do you believe your relationship with food and physical health is part of a spiritual battle? Why or why not?
- What would your ideal relationship with food look like? How would it affect your thoughts, eating habits, and lifestyle?

Breaking Habits & Overcoming Temptation

Many of our actions, behaviors, and choices are governed by habits. Even when we recognize bad habits, breaking them is difficult. Why is that?

Ask: Which of these reasons resonates most with you as to why breaking bad habits is so difficult?

- Long-standing habits feel comfortable.
- Some habits fulfill emotional needs.
- Some habits have become part of my identity.
- Immediate gratification is hard to resist.

Read Philippians 2:13

Ask: God is working in you, but you also have a role to play. What steps can you take to improve how you play your part in becoming the person God created you to be?

Physical Health & the Fruit of the Spirit

Read Galatians 5:22-23

Ask:

- How might greater energy, a stronger body, and a sense of vitality help you live out the Fruit of the Spirit (love, joy, peace, patience, kindness, goodness, faithfulness, gentleness, and self-control)?

- Could better health help you be more patient, joyful, or self-controlled?
- How might physical well-being contribute to your spiritual growth?

Replacing Lies with Truth

Read Proverbs 4:23

Ask:

- What are one or two lies or limiting beliefs you find yourself struggling with? Some examples include:
    - "I'm a failure; I'll never reach my goals."
    - "This is too hard; I give up."
    - "I deserve a treat because I had a hard day."
    - "I can eat whatever I want; it doesn't matter."
    - "I hate my body."
    - "This temptation is too strong; I might as well give in."

- How can you replace these lies with truths from God's Word?

Recognizing Satan's Lies About Food

Satan will do everything in his power to keep you from following the Holy Spirit's lead. He tempts you with choices that pull you away from becoming your best in God. His lies can have consequences in our health, self-worth, and spiritual growth.

Ask:

- What consequences have you faced from believing Satan's lies regarding food?
- How have these consequences affected your faith, health, and emotions?

Making Beneficial Choices

Read 1 Corinthians 6:12

Ask:

- In the week ahead, approach each food choice with this question: "I have the right to eat this, but is it beneficial?"

- Do you think some of your food choices might change if you consistently asked yourself this question?

Accountability Check-In (if pairing with the SoulStrength Fit Workout Program)

- Did you complete your workouts this week? What helped you stay on track, or what challenges made it difficult?
- How did you feel about your nutrition and eating habits this week? Can you think of a time when your choices reflected your goals—and a moment when it felt difficult to stay on track?

Closing Prayer & Prayer Requests

End the meeting with prayer, inviting members to pray for continued transformation, perseverance, and a deeper connection to God in all areas of their lives.

Looking Ahead

In the next session, members will discuss reflections from Week 2 of the devotionals. Encourage everyone to take notes on their experiences and insights gained throughout the week.

Session 3: Renewing Your Mind & Building Self-Discipline

Welcome & Opening Prayer

Begin by welcoming everyone and opening with prayer. Encourage members to pray for transformation and strength as they work toward aligning their health and fitness goals with God's plan.

Discussion: Breaking Free from Self-Sabotage

Read Romans 7:18-21 (The Message):

"If the power of sin within me keeps sabotaging my best intentions, I obviously need help! I realize that I don't have what it takes. I can will it, but I can't do it. I decide to do good, but I don't really do it; I decide not to do bad, but then I do it anyway. My decisions, such as they are, don't result in actions. Something has gone wrong deep within me and gets the better of me every time. It happens so regularly that it's predictable. The moment I decide to do good, sin is there to trip me up."

Ask:

- What habitual thoughts, feelings, or actions might you be accepting as normal, even though they hinder your growth or keep you from your deepest goals?
- How can submitting your health and fitness goals to God impact other areas of your life?

Transformation Through a Renewed Mind

Read Romans 12:1-2:

"Therefore, I urge you, brothers and sisters, in view of God's mercy, to offer your bodies as a living sacrifice, holy and pleasing to God—this is your true and proper worship. Do not conform to the pattern of this world, but be transformed by the renewing of your mind. Then you will be able to test and approve what God's will is—his good, pleasing and perfect will."

Ask: True transformation starts with a renewed mindset. How do you need to change your mindset in regard to your health and fitness? What thoughts, beliefs, or mindsets do you need to change?

The Importance of Self-Discipline

"Like a city whose walls are broken through is a person who lacks self-control." - Proverbs 25:28

Ask:

- In what specific areas or situations do you need to work on self-discipline?
- What's one area of your health or habits where you feel like you've been relying on your own emotions or willpower instead of God's strength? How might that be affecting your consistency or peace?
- Philippians 2:13 says that God works in us to ***will*** and to ***act*** according to His purpose. What's one example from this week where you felt God shaping your desires—or giving you strength to act on what's right?
- Can you think of a recent decision—big or small—where you had to choose between what felt good in the moment and what you knew would honor God? What did you choose, and what was the outcome?

- This devotional talks about buried emotions and past hurts that can influence present choices. Are there any emotions or thought patterns that might be influencing your habits more than you've realized?
- What does it look like in your life to "take every thought captive" when it comes to food, habits, or health choices? Are there any specific thoughts you need to replace with God's truth?
- The devotional compares your health journey to driving with headlights at night—just focusing on the next faithful step. What is one faithful step you feel led to take this week?

Accountability Check-In (if pairing with the SoulStrength Fit Workout Program)

- Did you complete your workouts this week? What helped you stay on track, or what challenges made it difficult?
- How did you feel about your nutrition and eating habits this week? Can you think of a time when your choices reflected your goals—and a moment when it felt difficult to stay on track?

Closing Prayer & Prayer Requests

End the meeting with prayer, inviting members to pray for continued transformation, perseverance, and a deeper connection to God in all areas of their lives.

About the Author

Kelly Wenner is the founder and creator of SoulStrength Fit and SoulStrength Fit Kids. With over two decades of experience in education, fitness, and spiritual development, Kelly is passionate about helping others deepen their faith and honor God in every aspect of life—including how they care for their bodies.

As a faith-based fitness expert and devotional author, Kelly's mission is to inspire and equip individuals to cultivate self-discipline, steward their health wisely, and recognize that caring for the body is an act of worship. Through SoulStrength Fit, she combines biblical wisdom with practical health and fitness strategies, creating programs and devotionals that encourage physical strength, spiritual growth, and wholehearted devotion to God.

Honoring My Temple reflects Kelly's heart for guiding others toward a healthier, more intentional life—one where faith and fitness are not separate, but beautifully intertwined. She prays this book will encourage readers to align their health choices with God's purpose, embrace self-discipline as a gift, and experience the joy and freedom that come from honoring their bodies in a way that glorifies Him.

Kelly lives in Southern California with her husband and three daughters, where she continues to find joy in serving others and sharing the transformative power of faith-centered health and wellness. To learn more about SoulStrength Fit, visit www.soulstrengthfit.com.

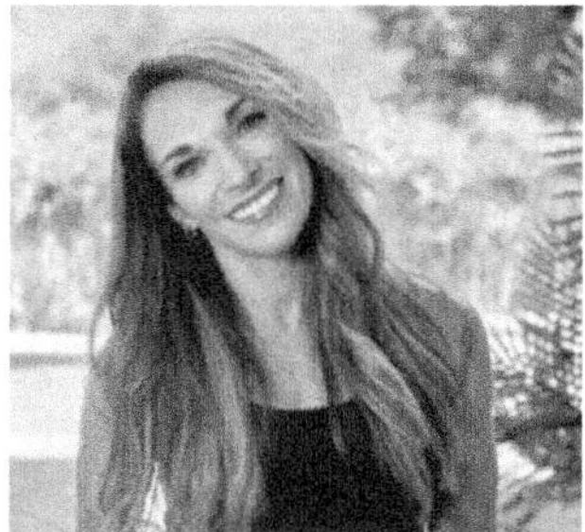